Patient Pictures

Rheumatology

by
John D Isaacs PhD MRCP, Senior Registrar in Rheumatology,
Addenbrooke's NHS Trust,
and Fellow, Downing College, Cambridge, UK

Series Editor
J Richard Smith MD MRCOG,
Senior Lecturer and Honorary Consultant Gynaecologist,
Charing Cross and Westminster Medical School,
Chelsea and Westminster Hospital, London, UK

Illustrated by
Dee McLean, MeDee Art, London, UK

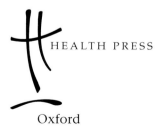

HEALTH PRESS

Oxford

Patient Pictures - Rheumatology

First Published 1995

© 1995 Health Press

25 Austin Place, Abingdon, Oxford OX14 1LT

A CIP catalogue record for this title is available from the British Library.

ISBN 1-899541-00-4

The author wishes to thank his colleagues at Addenbrooke's NHS Trust who
helped in the preparation of this book.

Copy editors: Amanda Klyne, Sarah Tarrant and Louise Walsh
Typeset by Laura Kinghorn
Designed by Design Online, Oxford, UK
Printed by Uniskill Ltd, Witney, UK

Contents

Reproduction Authorization

Author's preface

This book is for healthcare professionals to use with their patients. It aims to help them to prepare patients for their first visit to the rheumatologist and the treatments they may receive. Rheumatologists work as part of a multidisciplinary team with physiotherapists, occupational therapists and other healthcare workers. This team treats a variety of conditions, from sports injuries to osteoporosis and arthritis. Although some of these conditions are amenable to simple treatment such as a soft tissue injection, others may involve protracted care shared among the team.

It can therefore be very daunting and confusing for a patient attending the rheumatology clinic for the first time, particularly with a polyarthritis or multisystem disorder. What are the roles of the different medical staff? Why are there so many different forms of treatment? Some patients may wish to know how tennis elbow is dealt with, and how the injection is given. Others may be bewildered by the extensive examination they receive when all they have is painful hands; and who are the physiotherapist and occupational therapist? What are splints for?

Hopefully these words and pictures will remove some of the anxieties and maximize the benefit your patients receive from their first and subsequent visits to the rheumatology clinic.

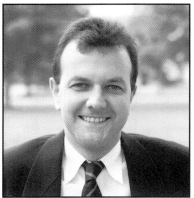

Louise Walsh

John D Isaacs PhD MRCP,
Senior Registrar in Rheumatology,
Addenbrooke's NHS Trust,
and Fellow, Downing College,
Cambridge, UK

Arthritis, the joints and surrounding tissues

- Joints are structures where bones meet. Healthy joints allow easy movement between the bones.

- Ligaments are tough white bands of tissue that hold the bones together at a joint. Muscles are the tissues that provide the power to move the joints. Tendons attach the muscle to the bone. Cartilage is a tough, slippery tissue that coats the end of the bones and prevents the actual bones rubbing together.

- Arthritis is inflammation of a joint, and leads to pain, stiffness and sometimes deformity. Although many joints may be affected at the same time, some forms of arthritis affect only one joint. Gout, for example, commonly affects just one big toe.

- 'Wear and tear' arthritis or osteoarthritis usually affects the weight-bearing joints: hips, knees and back.

- Rheumatoid arthritis – another common form of arthritis – often starts in the small joints of the hands and feet, but can affect any joint, including the neck and jaw.

- Less common forms of arthritis are associated with skin conditions such as psoriasis, or bowel disorders such as colitis. Others can follow infections, particularly viral infections, and gut infections which cause diarrhoea and food poisoning.

- Different types of arthritis require different treatments, and a major purpose of your visit to the rheumatologist is to allow the correct diagnosis to be made.

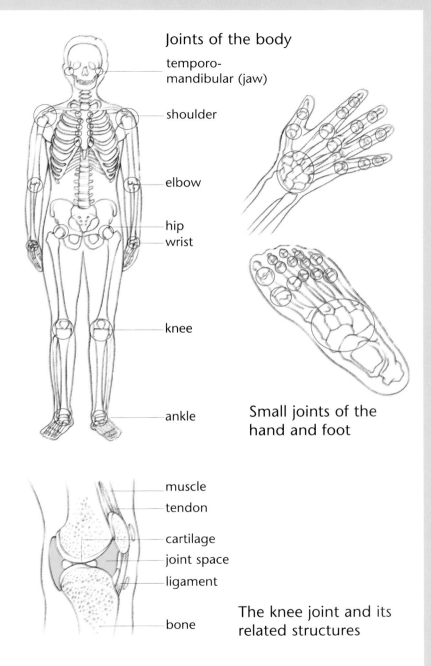

Joints of the body

- temporo-mandibular (jaw)
- shoulder
- elbow
- hip
- wrist
- knee
- ankle

Small joints of the hand and foot

- muscle
- tendon
- cartilage
- joint space
- ligament
- bone

The knee joint and its related structures

Arthritis and other body organs

- Some arthritic diseases can affect other organs as well as joints. Examples of organs that may be involved are the eyes, skin, heart, lungs, kidneys and nerves.

- An important aim of your visit to the rheumatologist is to find out if any other parts of your body are affected, as this will help the doctor to decide what is the best treatment for you.

- You may therefore be asked questions, for example, about rashes, chest or stomach pains, and pins and needles. In addition to examining your joints, the doctor may wish to listen to your heart and lungs with a stethoscope, examine your eyes, or palpate the area around your stomach.

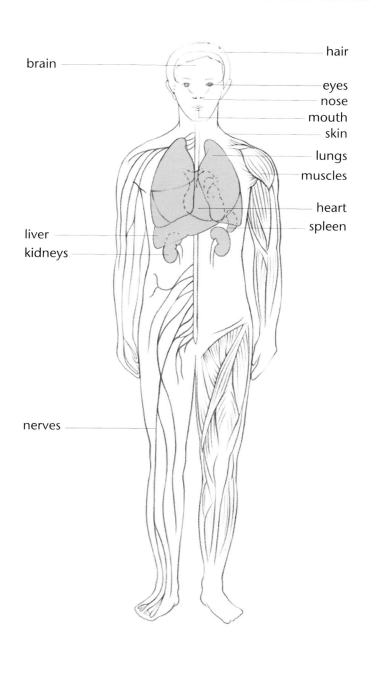

brain

hair

eyes

nose

mouth

skin

lungs

muscles

heart

spleen

liver

kidneys

nerves

Osteoarthritis

- Rheumatism is a general term used to describe pain in bones, muscles and joints. Arthritis is a disorder of the joints themselves, characterized by pain, stiffness and sometimes deformity.

- The two main kinds of arthritis are:
  – osteoarthritis ('wear and tear' arthritis)
  – rheumatoid arthritis (an inflammatory arthritis).

- In osteoarthritis, the joint cartilage (the tough, slippery tissue that usually coats the bones within the joint) gradually becomes worn down until the bones themselves rub against one another. This type of 'wear and tear' arthritis is more common in older people. Pain tends to be worse after activity, and at the end of the day.

- Pain-killers are commonly prescribed for 'wear and tear' arthritis. The mildest – paracetamol – may be sufficient to relieve pain. Stronger pain-killers often contain codeine and may cause constipation.

- If your pain is not adequately relieved by pain-killers, you may be referred to an orthopaedic surgeon. He will consider whether a joint replacement is likely to help you, and discuss this with you.

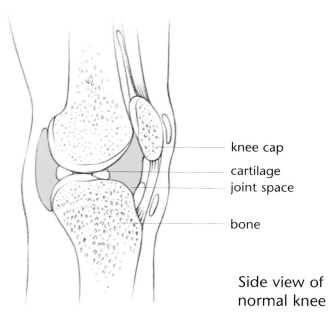

knee cap
cartilage
joint space

bone

Side view of
normal knee

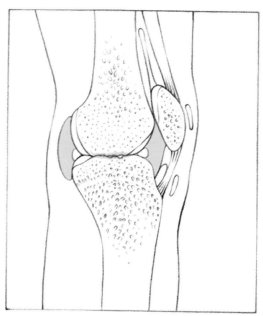

Osteoarthritis –
'wear and tear'
of the joint

Rheumatoid arthritis

- Rheumatism is a general term used to describe pain in bones, muscles and joints. Arthritis is a disorder of the joints themselves, characterized by pain, stiffness and sometimes deformity.

- The two main kinds of arthritis are:
  – osteoarthritis ('wear and tear' arthritis)
  – rheumatoid arthritis (an inflammatory arthritis).

- In rheumatoid arthritis, the tissues within and around the joints become inflamed, and the joints themselves become filled with fluid and white blood cells. The joints become red, hot, swollen, painful and stiff. The pain and stiffness are usually worse after periods of immobility (for example, first thing in the morning).

- There are a variety of drugs available to treat rheumatoid arthritis, including non-steroidal anti-inflammatory drugs (or NSAIDs), corticosteroids and what are called 'disease-modifying drugs'. As well as prescribing the appropriate medicine for you, your doctor may refer you to a physiotherapist, occupational therapist or other specialist to assist in your treatment.

- Occasionally, patients with rheumatoid arthritis are referred to an orthopaedic surgeon. Surgery may be necessary to remove severely inflamed tissue from a joint, or in some cases, to replace a badly damaged joint. The surgeon can also repair tendons that have become damaged as a result of inflammation, especially in the hand.

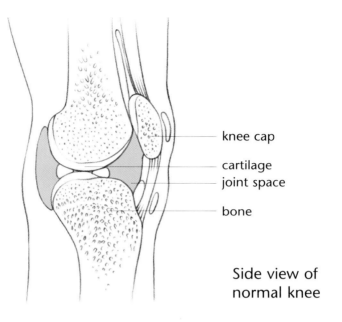

knee cap

cartilage
joint space

bone

Side view of
normal knee

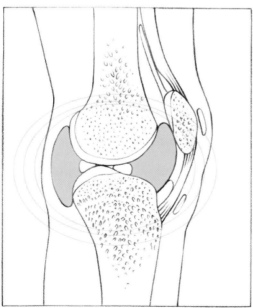

Rheumatoid
arthritis –
inflammation
of the joint

Monitoring arthritis

- Various measurements are necessary to monitor your arthritis and assess its response to treatment.

- The range of movement of a joint is a very important measurement. Minor reductions in movement resulting from inflammation or damage may be corrected with physiotherapy and occupational therapy, and therefore must be detected early on.

- When a joint becomes inflamed, the muscles moving that joint may waste (shrink and weaken). Simple measurement of muscle bulk (using a tape measure to measure around your thigh, for example) is a good indicator of muscle wasting and its response to treatment with physiotherapy.

- Various measurements can indicate the mobility of your spine, which is particularly important in inflammatory back disease. Examples are the distance between fingertips and floor on bending forwards or sideways.

- The change in the number of painful or swollen joints with time is an indication of response to treatment, as is the duration of 'morning stiffness'.

- Various scales may be used to measure your 'functional ability', such as the time you take to walk a certain distance or your ability to perform certain everyday tasks. You may be asked to fill in simple questionnaires with assistance from a doctor or nurse regarding your ability to cope with daily activities, level of pain, and general well being.

- Simple blood tests are also a guide to the level of activity of your arthritis.

Measuring elbow extension with a goniometer

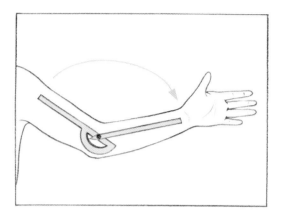

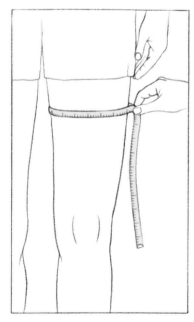

Measuring muscle bulk

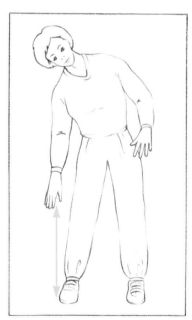

Measuring finger-to-floor distance

X-rays and other imaging investigations

- A number of imaging techniques are used in rheumatology. Imaging, which is like taking a picture of the inside of your body, helps the doctor to diagnose your problem.

- A standard X-ray shows the bony structure of the body. This is usually sufficient to distinguish different arthritic conditions, because inflammation and 'wear and tear' look different on the X-ray.

- Arthrography allows the doctor to see the 'capsule' surrounding the joint, and is particularly helpful in the diagnosis of shoulder complaints. It involves injecting a dye, which can be seen on the X-ray, into the joint before the X-ray is taken.

- A bone scan highlights areas of abnormal bone growth and joint inflammation. It is sometimes used when arthritis is suspected but X-rays are normal, and when inflammation of the spine is suspected.

- A CT scan takes several X-ray pictures at different points throughout the joint, rather like slices through a loaf of bread. It therefore shows the joint in more detail than a standard X-ray. CT scanning is commonly used to investigate back pain and sciatica when an operation is being considered.

- An MRI scan is similar to a CT scan, but is particularly good at highlighting injury to the 'soft' tissues, such as the ligaments, tendons and muscles.

- Having a CT or MRI scan involves lying still for up to 30 minutes within the scanner. Although some patients find being in the scanner a bit claustrophobic, it is not at all painful.

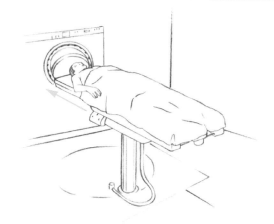

MRI scanner

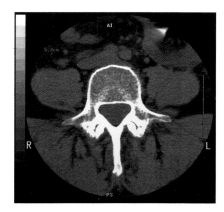

CT scan

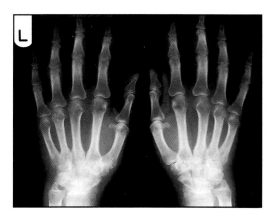

X-ray

Joint aspiration and injection

- Joint aspiration is the removal of fluid from a joint. This is particularly important in diagnosis when only one joint is inflamed, as it is the only way of finding out whether the joint is infected. If a joint is very swollen, aspiration may also relieve the pressure within the joint and thereby reduce pain.

- Sometimes, aspiration is followed by the injection of corticosteroid and local anaesthetic into the joint. The corticosteroid reduces inflammation, while the local anaesthetic relieves pain more quickly.

- Joint aspiration and injection are usually performed in the outpatient clinic. It is a good idea to rest the joint afterwards for one or two days.

- The joint and surrounding muscles should be resting and relaxed. The doctor will ensure that your joint is in a comfortable position.

- A needle is inserted into the joint. For most joints this is a very simple procedure, and local anaesthetic is not required. Joint fluid is aspirated (or sucked out) and, when required, corticosteroid and local anaesthetic are then injected through the same needle.

- The injection site may be covered with a plaster, which can be removed after about a day. You can have a bath or shower as there is no harm in getting the area wet.

- Sometimes the discomfort may worsen for the first day or so after an injection. Apart from this, there are usually no side-effects, but it may take several days before you feel a definite benefit.

- If the joint becomes extremely painful and swollen after injection, you should contact your family doctor straight away.

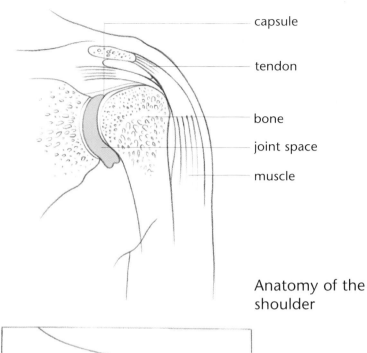

capsule

tendon

bone

joint space

muscle

Anatomy of the shoulder

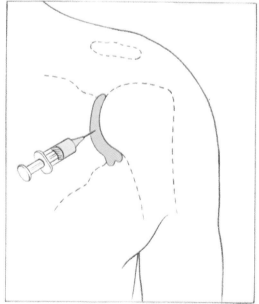

Injection/aspiration of the shoulder joint

Soft tissue injections

- Inflammation of the soft tissues – the ligaments, tendons and bursae – often responds to local corticosteroid injection.

- A bursa is a pocket of fluid lying between bone and skin, or bone and tendon, which prevents the bone from rubbing on, and damaging, adjacent structures. The lining of the bursa is similar to the lining of a joint and can become inflamed in the same way. A well-known example is housemaid's knee, which is due to inflammation of the bursa lying between the kneecap and the skin.

- The skin overlying the injection site is first cleaned with antiseptic. The injection is usually administered into, or close to, the tender area.

- Examples of soft tissue inflammation are tennis elbow and golfer's elbow, trochanteric bursitis (causing pain in the hip) and plantar fasciitis (causing pain in the sole of the foot).

- Tennis elbow and golfer's elbow result from inflammation at the sites where the forearm muscle tendons attach to bone.

- The trochanteric bursa overlies the bony prominence of the hip at the upper, outer thigh, and inflammation here causes trochanteric bursitis.

- The plantar fascia is the tough ligamentous tissue forming the sole of the foot. Plantar fasciitis is inflammation at its point of attachment to the bone beneath the heel, which causes pain on walking.

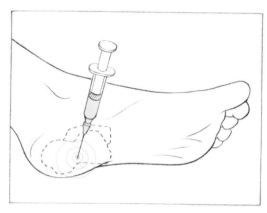

Injection for
plantar fasciitis

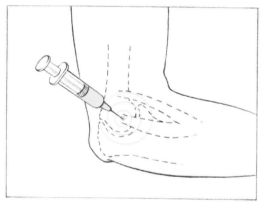

Injection for
tennis elbow

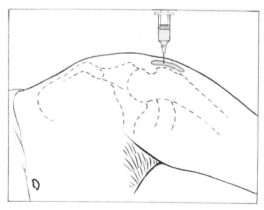

Injection for
trochanteric bursitis

Carpal tunnel syndrome

- Carpal tunnel syndrome is caused by pressure at the wrist on one of the nerves supplying the hand. It occurs where the nerve passes under a tight band of fibrous tissue. There is often no underlying cause for this problem, though it may occur in rheumatoid arthritis. It is also common in pregnancy.

- Symptoms are tingling and numbness in the thumb and adjacent fingers. Sometimes there is pain in the hand and arm, particularly at night. There may also be weakness of the thumb.

- Treatment usually involves an injection of corticosteroid at the wrist.

- Sometimes a splint is prescribed to relieve pressure on the nerve.

- Occasionally, an operation is required to relieve pressure on the nerve.

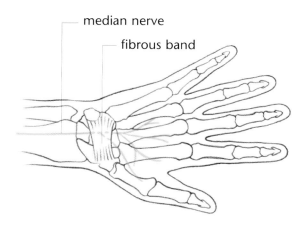

median nerve

fibrous band

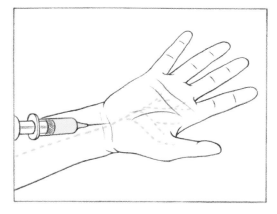

Injection for carpal tunnel syndrome

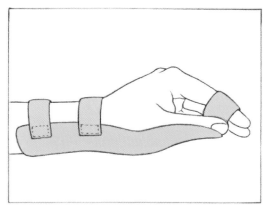

A splint for carpal tunnel syndrome

Electromyography (EMG)

- The electrical impulses produced by muscles and nerves are sometimes recorded to help diagnose damage to these structures.

- In muscle testing, a very fine needle is inserted into the muscle, and the contractions are recorded. The results can indicate whether or not there is muscle damage. The procedure may cause minor twitching, but is not painful.

- Nerve testing involves placing two probes on the skin at points along the course of a nerve. The nerve is stimulated with one probe, and a recording made of the subsequent impulse reaching the other probe. Damage to the nerve is indicated by abnormalities of this impulse.

- For example, to diagnose carpal tunnel syndrome, the muscles at the base of the thumb may be tested as above. Also the nerve supplying these muscles, and supplying sensation to the thumb and adjacent fingers, may be tested. The nerve will be stimulated on one side of the wrist, and a recording made on the other.

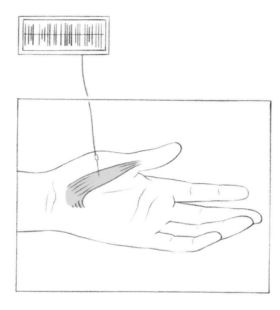

Testing muscle
function

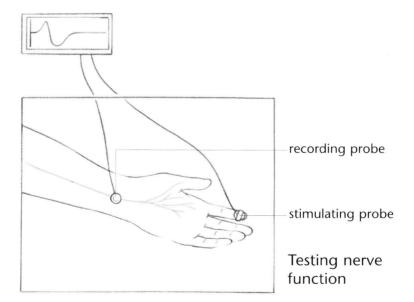

recording probe

stimulating probe

Testing nerve
function

Arthroscopy

- Arthroscopy enables the doctor to actually look inside the joint and may also be used for 'keyhole' surgery. Therefore, as well as assisting in the diagnosis of joint disease, it may also form a part of the treatment.

- Arthroscopy is commonly used to treat the knee, but can also be used for other joints.

- The procedure is carried out in a sterile operating theatre under general or local anaesthetic. With a general anaesthetic, you will be unconscious; if a local anaesthetic is used, your knee will feel completely numb but you will be awake.

- The arthroscope is a tiny 'telescope' which is inserted into the joint through a wider tube called a cannula. After the arthroscopy, there will be a small scar (less than 1 cm) where the cannula passed through the skin. There may be one or two other equally small scars, particularly if 'keyhole' surgery has been carried out. This allows the doctor to look through the arthroscope while the surgical procedure is carried out through a separate cannula.

- After an arthroscopy, local anaesthetic is injected into the joint to reduce any pain. It may be necessary to stay in hospital overnight, and occasionally longer.

- The joint should be rested for one to two days after an arthroscopy. The doctor will probably place a thick pressure bandage over the joint which is usually removed one or two days later. The stitches are removed after a few more days.

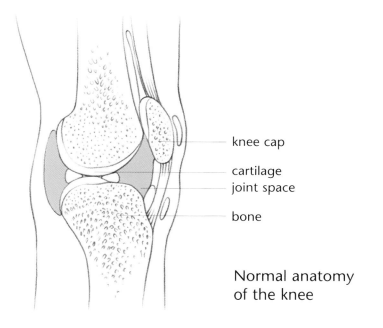

knee cap

cartilage
joint space

bone

Normal anatomy
of the knee

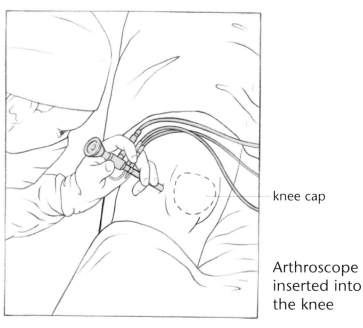

knee cap

Arthroscope
inserted into
the knee

Physiotherapy

- Physiotherapists are experts at joint rehabilitation and muscle re-education. They can also provide specific therapies for inflamed and damaged joints.

- In general, an inflamed joint should be rested. Exercise is crucial during the recovery phase to prevent the surrounding muscles from wasting and becoming weak. The physiotherapist will advise you on the best balance between exercise and rest.

- The physiotherapist can administer specific therapies to reduce the inflammation and pain of arthritis. These include simple measures such as ice packs to reduce swelling, or heat packs to ease pain. Other measures include ultrasound, and the provision of splints to ensure inflamed joints are rested in an appropriate position.

- Hydrotherapy involves exercising in a warm swimming pool. This enables joints to be exercised without stressing them too much.

- As joints recover, the physiotherapist will suggest graded exercises to gradually increase muscle strength.

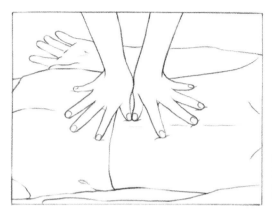

A mobilization technique to the lumbar spine

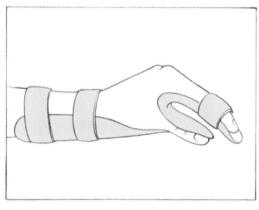

A 'resting' hand splint

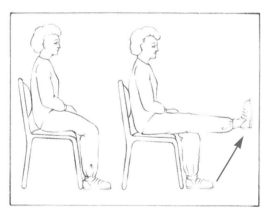

Quadriceps exercises (to build up the thigh muscles)

Hydrotherapy

- Hydrotherapy involves exercise in a warm swimming pool.

- Warm water assists relaxation of muscles and allows increased joint movement. Water also supports the joints and reduces the stresses on them during exercise.

- Only short periods of time are spent in the pool, usually between 10 minutes and half an hour.

- It is important to have a drink afterwards and to rest, because hydrotherapy can be very tiring.

- It is usual to have a course of supervised hydrotherapy treatment. Afterwards you may be given advice on exercises to perform on your own in your local swimming pool.

- You do not need to be able to swim to attend hydrotherapy. If you cannot manage steps, there is usually a lift to help you into the pool.

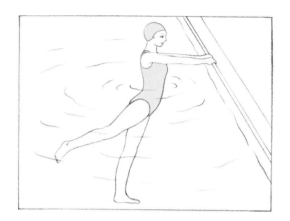

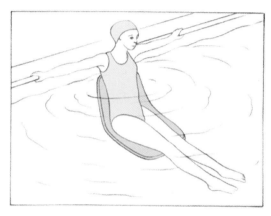

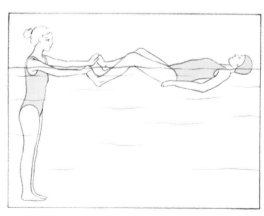

Exercises in the pool can be carried out in a variety of different ways, including free-standing, using equipment or with the help of a physiotherapist

Occupational therapy

- Occupational therapists are experts at joint protection and can teach you how to live with inflamed and damaged joints without making the damage worse.

- Occupational therapists are also skilled in assessing the function of weakened or damaged joints, and can provide help in making everyday life easier.

- The occupational therapist may supply gadgets to help you in the kitchen; for example, implements to help you to open tins, or to hold a knife and fork more easily. Other gadgets may help you to pick up items without bending down.

- The occupational therapist may recommend adjustments to your home, such as a rail to help you to get out of the bath, or higher chairs.

- Hand and wrist splints may be supplied by the occupational therapist. 'Working' splints protect your hands and wrists during daily life, and ensure an even distribution of forces across damaged joints, thus preventing further damage. 'Resting' splints are worn at night to prevent the development of deformities when your hands are resting.

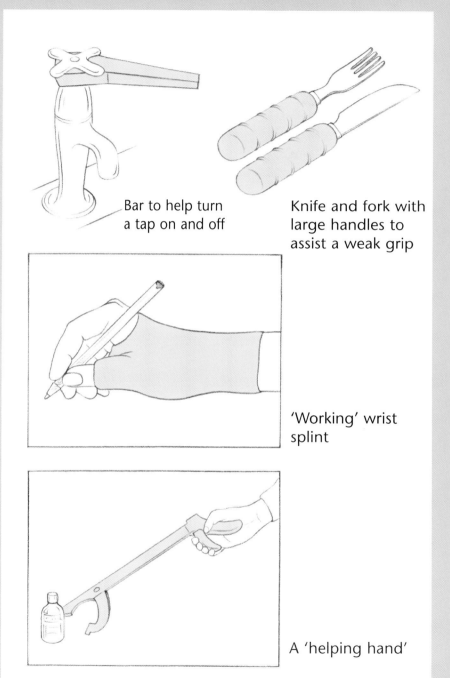

Bar to help turn
a tap on and off

Knife and fork with
large handles to
assist a weak grip

'Working' wrist
splint

A 'helping hand'

The orthotist

- The orthotist is skilled in assessing deformities and stresses across joints.

- When joints become damaged, the physical stresses across the joints that occur as a result of daily living may act to increase the damage and deformity. This is particularly true of the joints of the foot and leg.

- As with the hands and wrists, splints can be used to minimize the damage. This is more difficult in the feet, however, and the orthotist may make adjustments to shoes or design inserts to wear inside the shoes instead.

- Occasionally it may be necessary to have a pair of shoes 'made-to-measure'.

- The physiotherapist and orthotist may cooperate during the manufacture of other appliances, such as neck collars.

- With modern technology and materials, 'surgical appliances' or 'made-to-measure' footwear can be designed to blend in with your wardrobe.

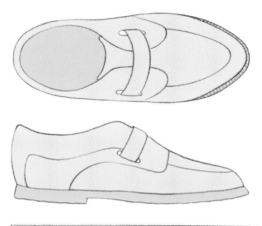

Made-to-measure
shoes

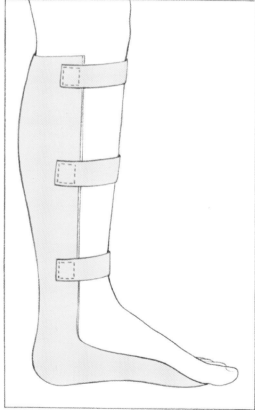

An ankle splint

The knee

- Pain in the knee can arise from arthritis of the joint or damage to the cartilage or ligaments within or around the joint. Damage to the cartilage or ligaments can occur with all types of arthritis, as well as following an injury, particularly from movements involving twisting. Inflammation can also occur in the pocket of fluid lying immediately in front of the knee – called the pre-patellar bursa – causing housemaid's knee. Arthritis of the spine or hip can also sometimes give rise to pain in the knee; this is called 'referred pain'.

- The events that occurred before the pain started, and the nature and exact location of the pain, will help the doctor to determine its origin. Examination of the knee involves not only bending and straightening it, but also movements that stress the tendons and ligaments. The back and hip may also be examined.

- Sometimes it may be necessary to aspirate fluid from the knee. This may be followed by an injection of corticosteroid and local anaesthetic. The corticosteroid reduces inflammation, while the local anaesthetic relieves pain more quickly.

- The needle may be inserted into either side of the knee.

- The knee should be rested for one to two days after an injection. During this time, the discomfort may worsen before it gets better. If the knee becomes extremely painful after an injection, and particularly if it becomes hot and swollen, you should contact your family doctor straight away.

- As the pain decreases following an injection, it is important to follow a regular exercise routine. You may be referred to a physiotherapist for advice on this.

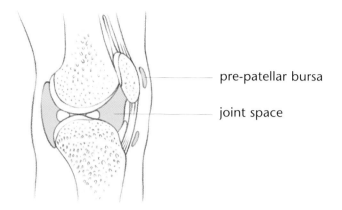

pre-patellar bursa

joint space

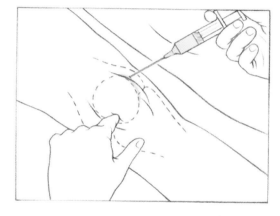

Aspirating and injecting the knee joint

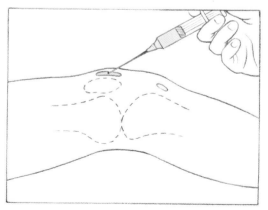

Aspirating and injecting the pre-patellar bursa

The shoulder

- Pain in the shoulder can arise from the joint itself or the surrounding structures – the capsule, tendons and ligaments. Inflammation of the capsule eventually leads to a 'frozen shoulder' with very restricted movement.

- Sometimes an injection may be necessary to relieve the pain. The needle may be inserted either into the shoulder joint itself or into the pocket of fluid called the subacromial bursa, which lies above the joint.

- Depending on the origin of the pain, the front, back or side of the shoulder may be injected with a corticosteroid and a local anaesthetic. The corticosteroid reduces inflammation, while the local anaesthetic relieves pain more quickly.

- Sometimes the discomfort may worsen for one to two days after the injection. If the shoulder becomes extremely painful after an injection, and particularly if it becomes hot and swollen, you should contact your family doctor straight away.

- As the pain decreases following an injection, it is important to follow a regular exercise routine. You may be referred to a physiotherapist for advice on this.

- Physiotherapy is particularly important for a frozen shoulder, which can take many months to heal.

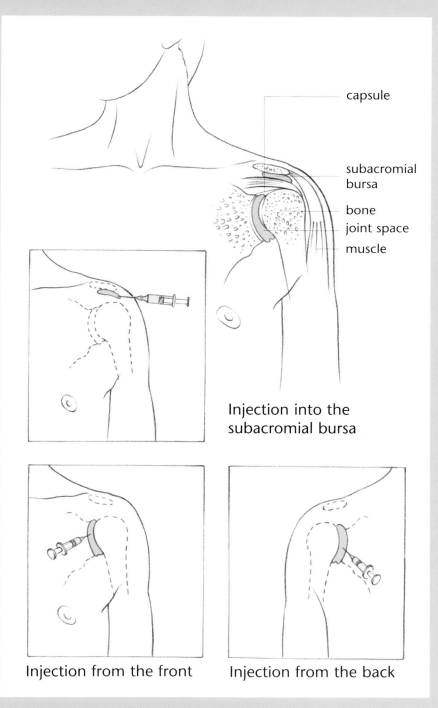

capsule

subacromial bursa

bone
joint space
muscle

Injection into the subacromial bursa

Injection from the front

Injection from the back

The wrist

- Pain in the wrist may arise from the wrist joint itself or from inflammation of the tendons overlying the joint (tenosynovitis). Tenosynovitis may arise from repetitive movements, but is also common in 'rheumatic' illnesses.

- Sometimes it may be necessary to aspirate fluid from the wrist. This may be followed by an injection of corticosteroid and local anaesthetic. The corticosteroid reduces inflammation, while the local anaesthetic relieves pain more quickly.

- The needle is usually inserted through the top or side of the wrist.

- Sometimes the discomfort may worsen for one to two days after the injection. If the wrist becomes extremely painful after an injection, and particularly if it becomes hot and swollen, you should contact your family doctor straight away.

- As the pain decreases following an injection, it is important to follow a regular exercise routine. You may be referred to a physiotherapist or occupational therapist for advice on this.

- Because the wrist is subjected to many stresses during daily use, it may be necessary to wear a splint, especially when the wrist is inflamed. This distributes forces more evenly across the wrist and prevents progressive damage to the joint. The splint will be supplied by your physiotherapist or occupational therapist.

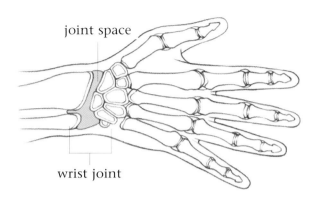

joint space

wrist joint

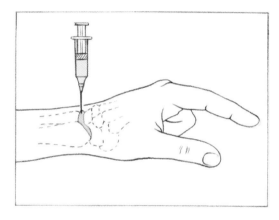

Injection into the wrist joint

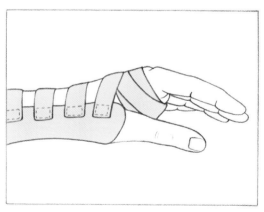

A wrist splint

The hand

- Pain in the hand may arise from the small joints of the hand or from inflammation of the tendons supplying the fingers (tenosynovitis). Tenosynovitis may arise from repetitive movements, but is also common in 'rheumatic' illnesses. It may be associated with a 'trigger finger'.

- Sometimes it may be necessary to inject one or two small joints, or the tendon sheaths, with corticosteroid to reduce inflammation.

- The joint at the base of the thumb is injected through the side of the hand at the wrist. Tendon sheaths are usually injected through the palm of the hand at the base of the fingers.

- Sometimes the discomfort may worsen for one to two days after the injection. If the joint or hand becomes extremely painful after an injection, and particularly if it becomes hot and swollen, you should contact your family doctor straight away.

- As the pain decreases following an injection, it is important to follow a regular exercise routine. You may be referred to a physiotherapist or occupational therapist for advice on this.

- Because the hand joints are subjected to many stresses during daily use, it may be necessary to wear a splint when the joints are inflamed. This distributes forces more evenly across the joints and prevents progressive damage.

- Deformities of the hand joints can also occur when the hand is resting, even during sleep. It is therefore important to wear night-time or 'resting' splints, which help to prevent such deformities.

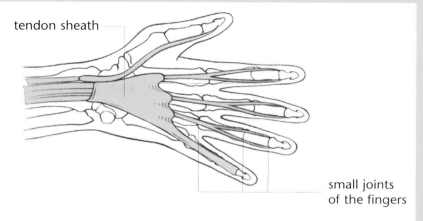

tendon sheath

small joints
of the fingers

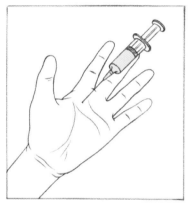

Injection of
tendon sheath

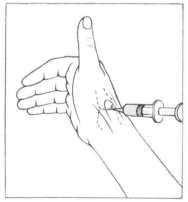

Injection into the joint at
the base of the thumb

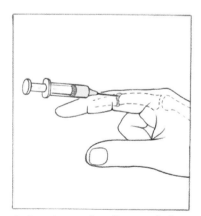

Injection of a finger joint

The foot

- Pain in the foot may arise from the small joints of the foot, or from damage to the tendons or ligaments. Damage to the tendons or ligaments may be the result of injury or inflamation. In arthritis, pain commonly arises from pressure on damaged joints during walking. Gout often affects the joint at the base of the big toe.

- Sometimes it may be necessary to inject one or two small joints with corticosteroid in order to reduce inflammation. This is necessary less often in the foot than in the hand.

- The needle is usually inserted through the side of the joint. Sometimes the discomfort may worsen for one to two days after the injection.

- If the joint becomes extremely painful after an injection, and particularly if it becomes hot and swollen, then you should contact your family doctor straight away.

- As the pain decreases following an injection, it is important to follow a regular exercise routine. You may be referred to a physiotherapist for advice on this.

- Because the foot and ankle joints are subjected to higher stresses during daily use than any other joints in the body, it is very important that they are protected properly. Modifications to shoes or inserts within shoes may be helpful. Common inserts are arch supports and metatarsal pads. As well as relieving pain, the aim is to prevent excessive forces across any particular joints that might increase the existing deformity. In some situations, you may be referred to an orthotist to have shoes or splints 'made-to-measure'.

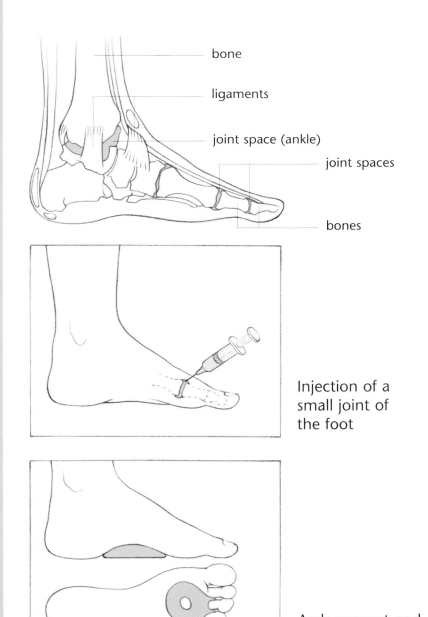

bone

ligaments

joint space (ankle)

joint spaces

bones

Injection of a small joint of the foot

Arch support and metatarsal pad

The elbow

- Pain in the elbow may arise from the elbow joint itself or from inflammation of the tendons adjacent to the joint (tennis elbow, golfer's elbow). Inflammation of the tendons may result from repetitive movements, but is also common in 'rheumatic' illnesses. The pocket of fluid (bursa) overlying the point of the elbow may also become inflamed (olecranon bursitis).

- Sometimes it may be necessary to take fluid from the elbow, or to inject it with corticosteroid and local anaesthetic. The corticosteroid reduces inflammation, while the local anaesthetic relieves pain more quickly. Similarly, a tennis or golfer's elbow may benefit from a corticosteroid injection.

- The needle is usually inserted through the side or back of the elbow for arthritis, or into the tender area at one or other side of the elbow for tennis or golfer's elbow.

- Sometimes the discomfort may worsen for one to two days after the injection.

- If the joint becomes extremely painful after an injection, and particularly if it becomes hot and swollen, then you should contact your family doctor straight away.

- As the pain decreases following an injection, it is important to follow a regular exercise routine. You may be referred to a physiotherapist for advice on this.

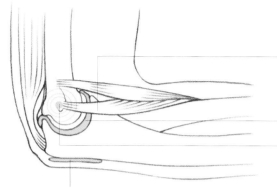

tendon

joint space

point of tenderness
in tennis elbow

olecranon bursa

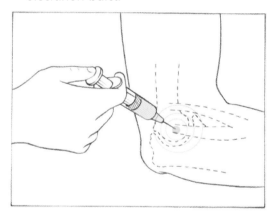

Injection of
tennis elbow

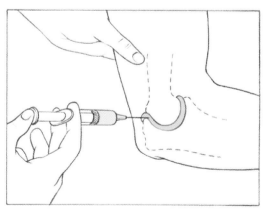

Injection of
elbow joint

The ankle

- Pain in the ankle may arise from the ankle joint itself or from damage to the ligaments and tendons surrounding the joint. Damage to the ligaments and tendons is usually the result of injury, particularly twisting movements. The Achilles tendon and adjacent bursae (pockets of fluid) may become inflamed in some rheumatic conditions.

- Sometimes it may be necessary to take fluid from the ankle, or to inject it with corticosteroid and local anaesthetic. The corticosteroid reduces inflammation while the local anaesthetic relieves pain more quicky. Occasionally, it is necessary to inject the bursae adjacent to the Achilles tendon.

- The ankle joint is usually injected from the front.

- Sometimes the discomfort may worsen for one to two days after the injection.

- If the joint becomes extremely painful after an injection, and particularly if it becomes hot and swollen, you should contact your family doctor straight away.

- As the pain decreases following an injection, it is important to follow a regular exercise routine. You may be referred to a physiotherapist for advice on this.

- If your ankle has been damaged by arthritis, there may be some deformity. Ordinary day-to-day walking may increase the stresses across the ankle and, under these circumstances, modifications to your shoes may be recommended. These are very important to prevent further pain and deformity.

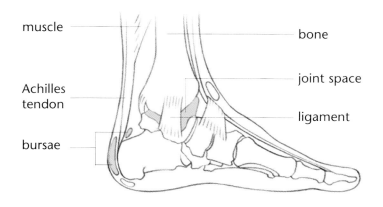

muscle

bone

joint space

Achilles tendon

ligament

bursae

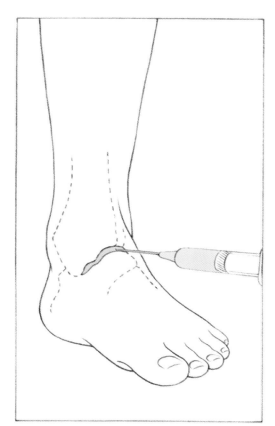

Injection of the ankle joint

The hips

- Hip pain is usually the result of 'wear and tear' arthritis, but the hips can sometimes be affected by an inflammatory arthritis or infection. Arthritis of the spine can also give rise to pain that appears to come from the hip, as can arthritis of the knee.

- Trochanteric bursitis is inflammation of the pocket of fluid (bursa) overlying the bony prominence of the upper, outer thigh. It is a common condition that often arises spontaneously, giving rise to pain in the outside of the hip.

- Sometimes it may be necessary to take fluid from the hip, or to inject the hip with corticosteroid and local anaesthetic. The corticosteroid reduces inflammation, while the local anaesthetic relieves pain more quickly.

- Trochanteric bursitis can readily be injected in the outpatient clinic. Unlike other joints, the hip is not easily accessible. Hip joints are therefore usually aspirated and injected in the X-ray department, using X-rays or ultrasound to guide the needle.

- The needle is usually inserted in the groin.

- Sometimes the discomfort may worsen for one to two days after the injection.

- If the hip becomes extremely painful after an injection, and particularly if it becomes hot and swollen, you should contact your family doctor straight away.

- As the pain decreases following an injection, it is important to follow a regular exercise routine. You may be referred to a physiotherapist for advice on this.

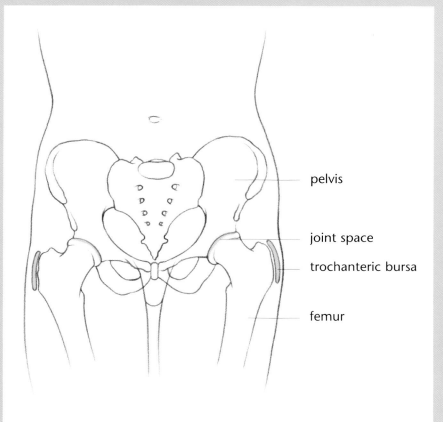

pelvis

joint space

trochanteric bursa

femur

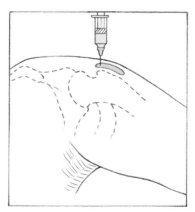

Injection for
trochanteric bursitis

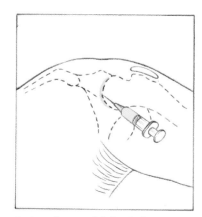

Injection of hip joint

The back

- Back pain, particularly lower back pain, is a major cause of ill-health. Lower back pain is often due to 'wear and tear' of the joints of the spine and is worse following activity, and eased by rest.

- Less commonly, the spine and its ligaments can be affected by inflammation (spondylitis). This results in stiffness after periods of rest. It can affect the entire length of the spine, as well as the sacro-iliac joints.

- In some cases, pain arises from the ligaments supporting the spinal bones. This is common in occupations involving a lot of standing or sitting, particularly if posture is poor. This is termed back 'strain'. Similarly, continued stresses affecting the sacro-iliac joints (in the lower back) result in sacro-iliac strain, with predominantly one-sided back pain.

- As well as examining your back, the doctor may give you a thorough examination to rule out less common causes of pain.

- Physiotherapy is a very useful treatment for all types of back pain. The exact form will depend on the nature of your problem, but may include exercises, traction (stretching of the back), hydrotherapy and local treatments such as heat and ultrasound. It is very important for correcting abnormal posture, relieving muscle spasm and rebuilding muscle strength. You may be encouraged to swim as this is an excellent form of exercise for back problems. Regular exercise is especially important for inflammatory back pain to prevent the development of back deformities.

- A firm bed and mattress may help to ease long-standing or recurrent back pain.

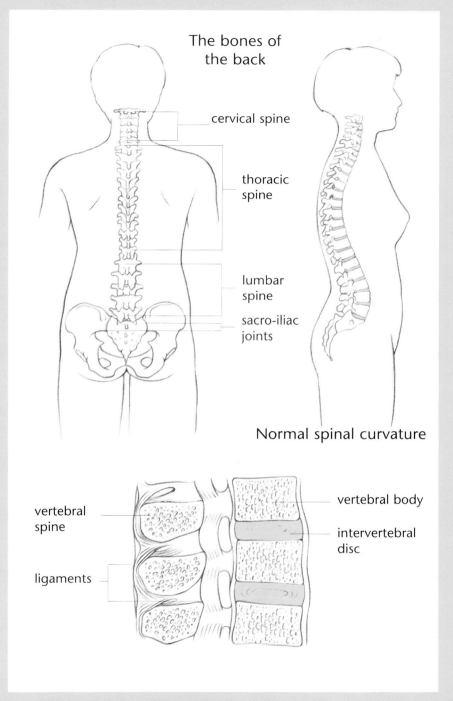

24

The bones of
the back

cervical spine

thoracic
spine

lumbar
spine

sacro-iliac
joints

Normal spinal curvature

vertebral
spine

ligaments

vertebral body

intervertebral
disc

'Slipped' disc

- Discs are packets of fibrous tissue that separate the individual bones that make up the spine (vertebrae).

- Excessive pressure or strain can cause a disc to 'give' and bulge out from between the vertebrae. This can result in pressure on nerves that run nearby. This, in turn, causes pain in the areas of skin served by these nerves.

- Slipped discs usually occur in the low lumbar spine, giving rise to pain in the back of the leg or 'sciatica'. Sometimes pain is felt at the front or side of the leg.

- As well as examining your back, the doctor will look for signs of nerve root irritation. This involves testing the sensation, power and reflexes in your legs. 'Straight leg raising' (where the doctor elevates your leg while you lie on the couch) stretches the sciatic nerve, and may mimic your 'sciatic' pain. The doctor may need to test the sensation of the skin around the back passage and genital area. Occasionally, the back passage will need to be examined internally.

- Most cases of sciatica improve with a period of lying flat in bed (for up to two weeks), after which there is a gradual return to normal activity.

- Sometimes physiotherapy is required to mobilize and re-educate the back.

- X-rays of the spine are occasionally taken. Scans are only necessary if rest and physiotherapy have failed to relieve the pain, and back surgery is being considered.

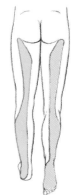

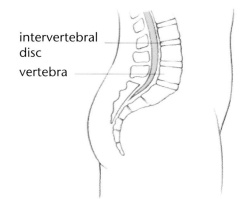

intervertebral disc

vertebra

Common location of 'sciatic' pain

The lower lumbar spine

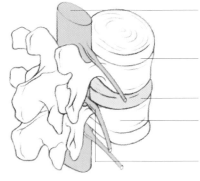

spinal cord

normal intervertebral disc

'slipped' intervertebral disc

vertebra

compressed nerve root

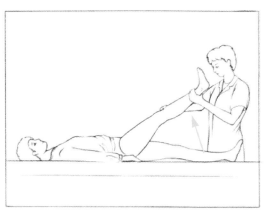

Testing 'straight leg raising'

Neck pain

- Neck pain is very common. It is usually the result of 'wear and tear' arthritis, but can also occur in rheumatoid arthritis. It may simply be due to poor posture.

- Occasionally, arthritis in the neck can result in 'trapped nerves' and this can cause tingling, pain and weakness in the arms and hands, or headaches. Rarely, neck arthritis can cause damage to the spinal cord. This may result in weakness of the legs as well as the arms.

- Assessment by the rheumatologist will include not only neck movements, but also an examination of your arms and legs. Sensation, strength and reflexes will be tested. An X-ray may be taken, but a scan is not usually necessary unless there are signs of significant nerve damage, and an operation is being considered.

- A combination of rest and physiotherapy relieves most cases of neck pain, and it may be necessary to wear a collar for a while to rest the neck by preventing excessive movements. It is also important to make sure your working environment is not causing problems; computer monitors, for example, must be at an appropriate level to prevent abnormal neck postures and your chair should support your back properly.

- Physiotherapy is helpful to reduce inflammation in the neck joints using physical treatments (for example, heat and ultrasound). Physiotherapists can also mobilize your neck when the muscles have become stiff and tight, as muscle spasm increases neck discomfort. Traction or stretching of the neck can be helpful when there are symptoms from trapped nerves.

- Most neck problems recover with these treatments. If symptoms recur, trigger factors should be looked for, particularly in the working environment.

26

Anatomy of the cervical spine

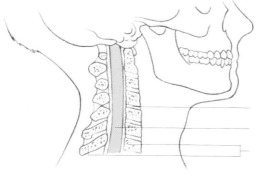

intervertebral disc
spinal cord
vertebra

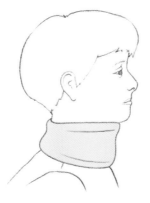

A cervical collar

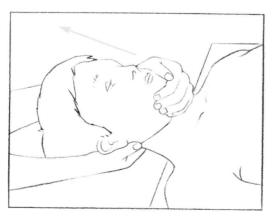

Cervical traction

Osteoporosis

- Osteoporosis (or thin bones) most commonly affects women after the menopause when oestrogen levels fall, because oestrogens (the female sex hormones) help to keep the bones strong.

- There are other risk factors for osteoporosis, such as heavy smoking or drinking, long-term treatment with corticosteroids, and surgical removal of the ovaries before the menopause. Osteoporosis also runs in families.

- The consequences of osteoporosis are numerous. You may develop severe back pain because there is a tendency for the vertebrae of the spine to collapse and become flattened. You may lose height and develop a stoop. You are also more susceptible to fractures, particularly of the hip and wrist.

- You may be referred to a rheumatologist for assessment of your bones. Standard X-rays or CT scans may be used to assess bone strength. In some hospitals, it is possible to have a formal 'bone density' assessment. This does not involve injections and is similar to having a standard X-ray of your back and hip.

- Osteoporosis is commonly treated with hormone replacement therapy (HRT), either as a pill, injections or skin patches. There are various forms of HRT, not all of which lead to a recurrence of your periods. There are also other forms of treatment if HRT is unsuitable, some of which must be given by injection, but a number are available as tablets. Regular exercise and a healthy diet are also important.

- A repeat bone density measurement may be taken after about a year to ensure that the treatment is working. Treatment is usually continued for many years and may be lifelong.

27

Common locations of fractures associated with thin bones

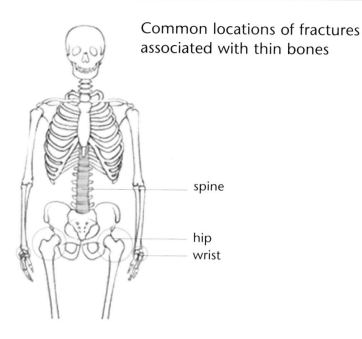

spine

hip
wrist

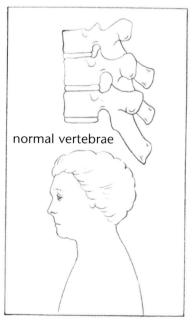

normal vertebrae

Normal spine

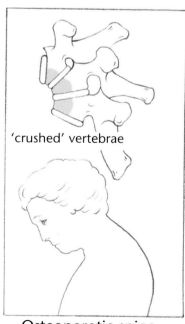

'crushed' vertebrae

Osteoporotic spine

Polymyalgia rheumatica

- Polymyalgia rheumatica is a common condition in the elderly, the cause of which is usually unclear.

- Polymyalgia rheumatica gives rise to severe pain and stiffness of the shoulder, neck and hip muscles and this is particularly severe first thing in the morning. It may be difficult to lift off the bedclothes or get out of bed, and you may feel generally unwell.

- Sometimes polymyalgia rheumatica is associated with inflammation of the arteries of the head and scalp (temporal arteritis), giving rise to headaches, scalp tenderness, visual disturbances, and pain in the jaw muscles on eating.

- Diagnosis may not be easy, but a blood test called the ESR may show a very high reading. In the case of arteritis, a tiny piece of tissue from one of the arteries running across your forehead (the temporal artery), may need to be taken. This is called a biopsy, and is performed in the operating theatre under general or local anaesthetic.

- Polymyalgia rheumatica is usually treated with corticosteroids which give rapid relief in one to two days. Treatment needs to be continued for one to two years, but after the first few months you will be taking only a small dose. The corticosteroid dose is gradually reduced to zero; sometimes the disease flares up again requiring a temporary increase. While taking corticosteroids, you should always carry a 'steroid card' which gives information about your medication. You should never stop taking corticosteroids suddenly.

- If there is an associated arteritis, the initial corticosteroid dose needs to be higher, and treatment is usually for longer.

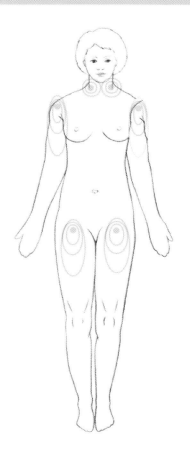

28

Areas of stiffness in polymyalgia rheumatica

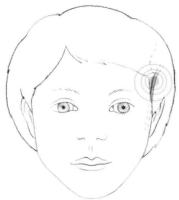

Area of headache and tenderness in temporal arteritis

Fibromyalgia

- Fibromyalgia is a common condition, particularly in middle-aged women. It causes generalized muscle and joint aches and pains, which may be associated with severe tiredness and sometimes depression. There is often a disturbed sleep pattern with a feeling of exhaustion on wakening. The cause is unknown, but it is not a serious or progressive condition, nor a sign of any underlying disorder.

- Diagnosis is difficult because there are no unique features, and all blood tests are normal. You may be tender over specific sites throughout your body.

- There is some evidence that a poor sleep pattern in this condition leads to a vicious circle of poor sleep, resulting in more aches and pains, worse sleep, and so on.

- You may be prescribed a small dose of an antidepressant to be taken at night. It is important to understand that this is not being given for its antidepressant properties, but because it can correct an abnormal sleep pattern and thereby help to relieve your symptoms.

- As your sleep pattern improves, you will be given a set of graded exercises to perform to re-establish muscle tone and power.

- It is important to understand that fibromyalgia is a real condition, and not something that is 'in the mind'.

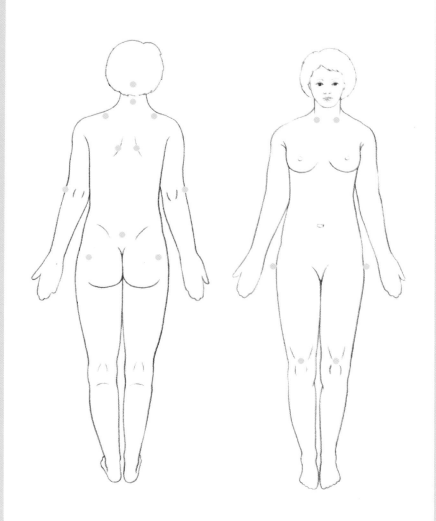

Tender sites in fibromyalgia

Mail Order

Patient Pictures – **Rheumatology** is the first book to be published in the *Patient Pictures* series. Forthcoming titles include Gynaecology, Prostatic diseases and their treatments, and Vascular surgery. Additional copies of this book are available at a unit price of £9.95 (post-paid in the UK only). Please send your name and address, quantity required, and a cheque for the appropriate amount made payable to 'Health Press' to:

Health Press
25 Austin Place
Abingdon OX14 1LT

Health Press titles are available at special discounts when purchased in bulk quantities for trusts, associations or institutions.

Please call our Special Sales Department in Abingdon on:

Tel: 01235 522147
Fax: 01235 528858